THE Cure Code

Discover the gift within you. 99% of your ancestors never had Cancer, Heart Disease, Diabetes or Obesity

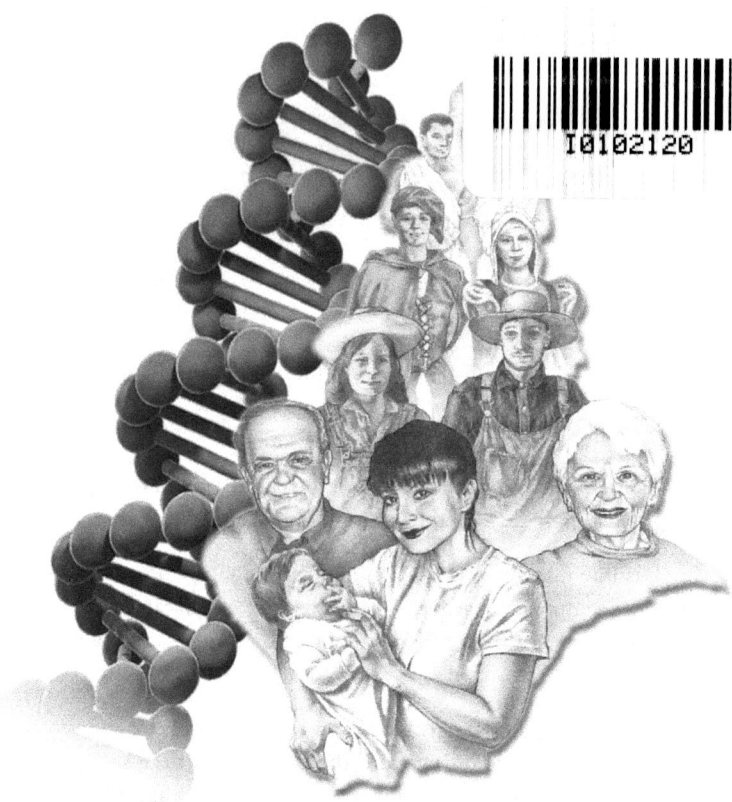

REGINALD L. FRANCISCO, R.PH

*This book is dedicated
in memory of my dad.*

Table of Contents

Foreword

Throughout history, man has looked to the heavens and stars for answers, but the answers may well be inside ourselves. Throughout time, man has only seen glimpses of the universe within.

Part of my mission in writing this book is to introduce new concepts and ideas.

One new concept may relate to a key that controls aging. One key of *The Cure Code* is that when this key is turned in one direction rapid aging occurs, and when turned in the other, the aging process slows down. Progeria Children Syndrome is an extremely rare and incurable genetic disease that causes premature, accelerated aging. Progeria ages the body rapidly, leaving teens (8–15) with frail, 80- to 90-year-old bodies and causes early death. One special dietary component may provide a key to living a long, healthy life. Essentially, children with Progeria lose this component and the genetic key is turned forward, making them look like old people.

What these children lost, these people found. The long-lived, healthy Japanese villagers and Okinawans who eat this special component as the core of every meal live long, healthy lives. In fact, they turned the key backward and in doing so they have the longest disability-free life expectancy in the world. They also have the highest percentage of centenarians (people over 100) anywhere on earth. The theory is this component cocoons the cells and prevents disease. One more fact I'd like to mention, is that these women, in their 90s, have almost no wrinkles in their skin. We will investigate these phenomena in detail.

How long would you like to live? Would you like to remain healthy and active even in your *golden years?* Does this sound like a dream?

The Cure Code will help individuals understand that as we changed the nutritional time line in which we began to eat foods that mankind had never eaten before such as refined sugar, refined flour, rice and potatoes, we changed the genetic time line and it caused us to acquire serious diseases that we never had before. Approximately one million of your ancestors (which is about 99%) never had cancer, heart disease, or diabetes and were never overweight.

Walk down the halls of any large hospital and you will probably see signs reading: Cardiology, Child Physiology, Clinical Pharmacology and Toxicology, Endocrinology, Gastroenterology, Hematology/Oncology, Immunology, Neonatology, Neurology, Rheumatology, Gynecology, Urology, Hematopathology, Microbiology, and Pathology. But something is missing. Why don't we see a sign for **Preventology** *to protect us in advance from all these possible illnesses so we can have a prolonged, healthy life?*

More and more of us are watching our weight and trying to diet, and we plan to exercise more often if only we could find the time. As we struggle to be *healthy,* many of us sometimes wonder if it's all worth it. As my Aunt Nelly used to say, "We should just enjoy all those fried foods and delicious desserts— since everyone just gets old, sick and dies anyway."

But isn't the quality of life as important as its quantity?

Today, in fact, a growing number of doctors and scientists would argue with my Aunt Nelly. Their research seems to indicate that if we maintain a healthy lifestyle, *eating for life*, our bodies stand a good chance of aging more slowly and more gently, without suffering the diseases people have come to associate with later life, such as stroke, heart disease and cancer. Eating organic, unprocessed foods low in sugar and fats—and exercising regularly—help us look and feel better. And most important, proper diet enables us to take advantage of the support that our genetic memory—the most powerful force on earth—offers to each one of us.

In this book, we will focus on *health* fitness, not *physical* fitness. Even diet gurus like Dr. Robert C. Atkins and fitness gurus like Jim Fixx did not live especially long lives despite all their diet and physical fitness efforts and advice. Dr. Atkins died in 2003 at age 72, and Jim Fixx passed away at age 52 in 1984. Lifestyle is important and all-encompassing; it is not just about *dieting* or *running*. We need to take advantage of the genetic gift our ancestors left us. A *healthy* lifestyle has to be one that most people can follow comfortably and easily each day as they go about their daily lives.

And on an individual level, this book is about hope. I want first to empower you and show you what you can do for yourself today. Then, together, we will explore what science and medicine can do for all of us in the future as researchers learn more about our DNA and how it has worked to produce the greatest force in our physical lives—our genetic intelligence.

With *The Cure Code* you can empower yourself. You can create and develop your own internal makeover—a makeover that will help you prevent disease and create a balanced, productive and stable lifestyle using tools currently available to anyone.

Let's begin!

A Personal Note from the Author

This book is about saving lives and improving health.

Although I am not a medical doctor, as a registered pharmacist I have worked in some of the most respected hospitals in the United States. At Walter Reed Army Medical Center in Washington D.C., I worked as an Inpatient Pharmacist. At The Johns Hopkins Hospital in Baltimore, Maryland, I was an Intravenous Products Pharmacist. I also worked as a Patient Care Pharmacist with The Johns Hopkins Health Care System in Baltimore. While serving as a Lieutenant in the United States Navy, I was the Director of a Pharmacy Medical Clinic in Philadelphia, Pennsylvania. I hold a Bachelor of Science degree in Pharmacy from Ohio Northern University in Ada, Ohio, and I am licensed as a Registered Pharmacist in the states of Ohio and Pennsylvania.

Every day in my work as a pharmacist I witness millions of dollars being spent on medicines and treatments. Why this emphasis? Because western medicine still focuses on *treating* illness rather than on *preventing* it. There is a wealth of information available that has been shown to help people take control of their own health, but few have yet tried to bring it together in one place and make it easy for *you* to find and use.

In this book I will bring much of this information together for you because I want to give you hope and empower you to have a hand in your own health and the health of your family.

First of all, there is a great deal you can do for yourself that doesn't cost a great deal of time and money. I will introduce *Preventology,* a new concept, which can save you a considerable amount of money in doctor bills and insurance premiums.

In doing the research for this book, I began to notice a fascinating link connecting various things I was learning—an organizing principle, if you will. I came face-to-face with this powerful notion during a severe attack of food poisoning. I now know this is a conscious and intelligent force. It saved my life. I call it "Genetic Intelligence," and I want to share this groundbreaking personal discovery because I have come to believe that Genetic Intelligence is accessible to everyone, enormously powerful, and incredibly easy to understand and to apply in your life.

"Preventology" will help you to learn the diet and health habits that will enable you to work with your own very personal genetic intelligence in such a way as to support you and help you prevent disease, improve your health, and prolong your life.

The Preventology concept springs from ideas that are natural. They are not new. Nature has been testing them for millions of years. As we go along you will see how to partner with the genetic intelligence you inherited from your earliest ancestors and use it to enjoy a longer, healthier life.

I want to thank all the fine authors and researchers who are adding precious knowledge to what we now know about maintaining and improving our health. Many of their ideas have been included in this book. Please refer to the list of sources in the back of the book if you would like to explore their work in more detail.

—Reginald L. Francisco, R.Ph

Introduction

This book intends not only to inform you but also to provide new tools to help you lead a longer, healthier life. My goal is to show you a pattern of events and ideas that will introduce you to a distinct force or consciousness that lies within everyone—in our genes.

What is Genetic Intelligence?

We all possess what appears to be a hard-wired genetic intelligence, which at most times we are completely unaware of—except for what we often call "instinct," like the fight-or-flight reaction we encounter when surprised or threatened.

A developing medical theory of genetic memory states that it is possible to uncover within ourselves a deep but accessible memory imprinted upon our genetic make-up as a result of what our ancestors experienced. This information is thought to be stored in your DNA (deoxyribonucleic acid) in a way that geneticists are just beginning to understand.

With healthy eating habits and sensible exercise, along with your genetic programming, it is possible to take advantage of the power of genetic intelligence.

Why should you care about genetic intelligence?

Let's start with your future—your children. If you and your family have developed poor eating habits and carry on a lifestyle that lacks exercise—a very common phenomenon in the U.S. these days—you and your children are at risk for major health problems at any age. We are seeing the signs of that danger today.

For example: A diabetes epidemiologist at the Centers for Disease Control and Prevention warns that one in three U.S. children born today will become diabetic (Type II adult-onset) unless we change our dietary habits. He adds that nearly half of all black and Hispanic children are likely to develop the disease. Diabetes, of course, can lead to blindness, kidney failure, and amputation of limbs and may also encourage or hasten the onset of heart disease.

An article published in the *American Journal of Pathology* states that all children who consume the rich western diet (i.e., the all-too-typical American high fat, high sugar, high carbo-hydrate diet) tend to show early signs of atherosclerosis (artery damage caused by fatty streaks)—often by the age of three! This inexorably leads to the early stages of heart disease, and it can all begin while a child is still a toddler.

According to the American Dietetic Association, obesity rates in the U.S. have doubled for adults and tripled for school-age children and adolescents over the past several decades. One child in three is now overweight or obese. These are, of course, the prime candidates for Type II diabetes and eventually for heart disease. Many obese children also develop chronic orthopedic problems, and increasingly they are being found to suffer from liver diseases and asthma.

In fact, these problems—all of them—are reaching epidemic proportions. What is the solution? It's *The Cure Code*.

Christopher Columbus was told the world is flat and he could not cross over the edge; he would fall off! Like Columbus, medical science today says that you are already genetically at risk for certain diseases and will probably die at around age 78. Columbus crossed that line and discovered a new world. I invite you to do the same. I invite you to come with me on a voyage of discovery to learn how to work with an intelligent force that has existed in your genes for perhaps 600 million years—a force that can bless you and your children with good health and a longer life.

Along the way, we will examine *anomalies*, one of the most promising areas for new discoveries. Anomalies are exceptions to the way things usually work. They show us new possibilities, and science can make major progress by studying them. We will also look at what science and medicine are doing today and suggest some promising new avenues for future research.

While today's genetic research may take years to produce information that you can use to improve your health and live longer, *you* don't have to wait. We will finish this part of our voyage by introducing you now to one of the core concepts of this book. **Preventology** will show you how to use simple, inexpensive, natural methods that work with your powerful genetic intelligence to promote good health now.

Nutritional Genetics is an emerging new science that has been developing rapidly over the last ten years. Fundamentally, it is the interplay between nutrition and genes.

Ninety-nine percent of your ancestors never had cancer, heart disease or diabetes and were never overweight. The holy grail of health lies in understanding this interplay as part of *The Cure Code*.

We would like to see that become the norm once again, and this book is just a beginning, a "first step" to helping you develop your own workable, personal version of *The Cure Code*.

Chapter 1—
Your Genetic Intelligence

What are Genes?

If you could see the microscopic DNA in your cells, each strand would appear much like a double spiral staircase. In the book *Grow Younger, Live Longer,* doctors Deepak Chopra and David Simon remind us that DNA has remained much the same for the last 600 million years. Chemically, DNA is not glued together any more firmly than a leaf or a speck of pollen, but it is resilient. It has survived in spite of powerful forces, and its powerful inner intelligence has defied time and the elements for ages. Moreover, it has changed as our species has changed and evolved, and those changes are what we must aim for as we re-define the concepts of "health" and "wellness" in this age of mankind (for the benefit of those yet to be born as well as, in this life, for ourselves).

Genes are lengths of DNA that were transmitted from your parents to you, half from your mother and half from your father, and which, in its newly combined form, passes on to your children. Genes make up only about three percent of the *6000 million* base pairs of DNA in almost every one of your cells. Genes give us characteristics, or traits. Scientists believe that ancient people who inherited traits that helped them to survive and reproduce better than others were more likely to procreate and to pass on healthy, strong genes to their children.

Alterations or mutations in the DNA sometimes produced new traits. Most of the mutations were damaging in some ways and eventually disappeared because those who carried them were less likely to survive or reproduce. However, some mutations helped their carriers survive even better, and these were then passed on to their offspring.

Your Genetic Heritage

In her book, *The Origin Diet,* Elizabeth Somer, M.A., R.D., describes the lifestyle of your healthy stone-age ancestors and suggests ways to modify your diet so you can enjoy better health. It's true that your genetic programming is based upon the habits of your ancestors. *Modern* diets, she notes, are a very recent development.

Eons ago, and even until recent centuries, the human diet consisted primarily of wild game and plants. Because they had no other choice, your healthy ancestors consumed a low-carbohydrate, calorie-restricted diet. Your ancestors were what historians and anthropolgists have called "hunter-gatherers." This way of life required extensive exercise—all day, every day. Because they lived only on what they could grow or kill, they spent most of their waking hours on the move, hunting game and consuming several pounds of vegetables, nuts, seeds and fresh fruits each day. Although diets varied based on geographic location and geological environment, researchers have concluded that a typical diet for your ancestors consisted (on average) of about 65 percent vegetables, fruits, seeds and nuts—all of which were, by definition, non-processed foods. They ate no refined sugars or hydrogenated fats. The rest of the diet consisted of wild game that was low in saturated fats and high in polyunsaturated fats (the good kind)—as opposed to today's farm-bred animals, which are force-fed to become fat and chemically treated in ways which are not always human-friendly (added hormones, for instance, can cause many medical conditions in those who eat processed meats, poultry and dairy products).

Study after study shows that the diet of most of our ancestors prevented obesity and heart disease and promoted good health. Scientists who have studied your ancestors' remains have verified without question that nutritionally, they lived healthy lives, and their remains show little or no evidence of having suffered from the diseases we have today. *Degenerative* diseases such as cancer, stroke, and heart attack were unknown. Our ancestors were, for the most part, as physically fit as today's athletes, and those who lived beyond their normal life spans remained active and relatively disease free. The primary causes of death in those times were accidents, battle wounds, and starvation. If their living environments had been safer, a bit more technologically advanced, and less harsh, they would probably have lived nearly as long as we do now. Stated in the simplest of terms, your ancestors gave you the gift of good health to enjoy—but only if and when you bring your lifestyle into harmony with your genetic blueprint.

Today your genes are almost identical to those your ancestors had some 40,000 years ago. So it makes logical sense to observe that when you emulate your ancestors' lifestyle with healthy eating and adequate exercise, you are supporting the genetic structure you have inherited from them and can thus enjoy the same good health and long life.

In generations past, people ate one food at a time as it became available to them—fruit from a tree, berries from a bush, root vegetables that grew wild. They didn't have a wide choice of combination meals like those on your plate today. Moreover, your ancestors weren't assured of daily meat consumption, either. Often, hunters would literally run for days to catch one small animal. This kept the pursuers lean and fit, and the animal they caught and ate provided them with lean meat because those animals got plenty of exercise, as well, as they ran for simple survival. A successful hunt was cause for celebration. People united, cooked their meat, and savored every precious bite. As a result of these eating patterns, the digestive system evolved in such a way as to work best (for you, today) when you eat the right kinds of foods and eat your foods slowly. Today, cooking the types of foods that your ancestors thrived on and then sitting down to a communal meal is a lost art. It's no wonder so many of you experience heartburn and indigestion after a hurried meal of sugar-laden, fatty foods at a fast food restaurant!

The kinds of foods your ancestors ate—both in terms of content and balance—also protected them from many diseases. They consumed *twice or three times as many fresh fruits and vegetables* as the average American eats today. In addition, their diet was rich in antioxidants, fiber, and many, many natural compounds that helped their bodies resist disease and prevent conditions like osteoporosis (bones that become porous and break easily because of calcium deficiencies in the diet). Your body still has this natural programming built into its genetic structure, and with proper attention to your individual and family diet you can realize many of the same benefits your ancestors enjoyed, including healthy outcomes like lower blood pressure and less risk of developing cancer and osteoporosis.

Remember that your healthy ancestors consumed only organic foods. If you choose to increase the amount of produce in your diet, it's a good idea to try to choose organic foods—foods that are grown or raised naturally and do not contain or harbor chemicals such as pesticides. By the way, always wash all produce thoroughly, whether organically grown or not, before you eat or cook it, since even most organic farmers today use manure as one of their main fertilizers, and this can contain harmful bacteria.

Here's something else to think about. Today's bumper harvests have come at a high price. The pesticides we use in conventional agriculture are poisonous to living organisms (pests), and their harmful effects on our bodies accumulate as we consume foods that have been treated with them. Government standards on *acceptable* levels of pesticides in foods are set to tell you how toxic *a single compound* is, but you and I are exposed to multiple pesticides every day—from conventional agriculture, from the water we drink, and in the air we breathe. Science and medicine don't know how much of this toxic load our bodies can safely handle.

Some researchers believe that people can avoid too many pesticides by genetically engineering their crops to resist pests. Genetic engineering, however, is a delicate process of taking genes from other plants, animals, or insects and putting these genes into the plants used for food. Since this has never happened in nature, researchers don't know what will happen to people who eat genetically engineered food for a long time or how it might someday affect those with allergies.

In the United States, staple foods like corn and soybeans are already being genetically engineered. And such conventional foods do not have to list any genetically engineered ingredients on their labels. The good news, though, is that certified organic foods are not allowed to include any genetically engineered ingredients.

You can easily recognize and appreciate the benefits of eating in the ways your ancestors did if you look at what happens when people in "primitive" cultures—whose diet resembles that of your ancestors—join the *modern* world and adopt its dietary habits. Studies done with modern-day hunter-gatherer tribes like the Aborigines in Australia show that prior to making fundamental dietary changes these people enjoyed excellent health and modern diseases were unknown. Two or three generations after the Aborigines started eating a *modern diet,* though, their rate of disease became virtually the same as the American statistics. When your diet and exercise patterns go against your genetic intelligence, you are fighting the greatest power on earth—your genetic memory—and you lose!

What is Genetic Memory?

Recently, a controversial idea has emerged, based upon the notion that our long-term memories may be passed on to and stored in our genes. Much work is being done in this area, but results are, by the very fact that they are at least generational, slow to show up in the real world.

Most neuroscientists still maintain that long-term memories are accumulated in our brains when connections between neighboring neurons are built and strengthened as we repeat behaviors and develop habits. These neural connections are known as synapses, and they connect neurons together to form complex networks that can recreate specific patterns of activity in our brains daily—or even years later. These patterns of brain activity, they say, give us our memories, and all that goes away when we die.

On the other hand, researchers who postulate that our memories may be added to and stored in our genes point out that for the synapse theory to be true the connections which synapses form would somehow need to be permanent and stable.

However, nearly all the molecules in the brain are replaced every few weeks, so it seems to be nearly impossible to store long-lasting memories in something that keeps changing. One adaptive theory says that the brain retains a blueprint of each neural network so it can create a replacement neuron that is structurally and functionally the same, replicating exactly the molecular structure and content it is replacing. When this idea is thought through, it becomes quite possible that the best choice for handling and storing this blueprint is DNA.

- Fact 1: DNA is stable and isn't replaced over time like other molecules, and
- Fact 2: it also can repair itself if anything goes wrong. If this is true, then our genetic code is quite likely not totally fixed at the beginning of our lives and can be altered a bit by interactions with our brain cells.

This concept of storing memory in our DNA raises some interesting questions. If we pass our DNA on to our children and they pass it on to their children, could this explain what happens when someone remembers a past life during past life regression? Is this individual actually accessing an ancestral experience that is present in his or her genomic blueprint? Also, if our memories are stored in our DNA, which is then passed on to future generations, could this also explain *instinctive* behavior like that of baby chicks that run from the shadow of a hawk even though they have never seen one before?

Besides the benefits you can reap by following the eating and exercise patterns of your ancestors, there are instinctive behaviors that you take for granted that have been passed down to you biologically for generations. Through evolution, your genes certainly seem to carry important information to be remembered for survival. These memories are passed on to you at birth, and this genetic information is passed down through DNA.

It is generally accepted by scientists in many disciplines that the human body retains a genetic memory of foreign substances it has been exposed to. An example is food poisoning. Food poisoning can be horrific and sometimes deadly. Microscopic organisms that cause food-borne illness are everywhere. Most grow undetected because they don't produce any unusual odor, color or texture in food. By some process not clearly understood, when we are exposed to toxic elements in food, most of the time we do not experience active food poisoning; our bodies are equipped to overcome it in a very natural and sometimes even unfelt way, protecting us against this threat to life and health.

The Power of Genetic Memory—Up Close and Personal

I have experienced the protective force of my genetic memory. It literally saved my life.

Several years ago, a friend and I were enjoying a leisurely vacation on a Caribbean island. At dinner one evening, she and I joked about how we had ordered the same meal, but I had decided to try an additional dish. Later that night, I was jolted from sleep by the most powerful systemic upset I've ever experienced. Being a pharmacist and a runner, I am physically fit. I'm very familiar with the effects of food poisoning, but this experience was different. I did not have the typical abdominal cramps that can be observed when running. The pain was different and lasted for hours. There was urgency about the whole process, as if something inside me knew I had to get this poison out of my system or I was literally going to die. After twelve hours of almost continuous and very severe vomiting, it was obvious to me that my body was violently attempting to expel the poisons from my system.

I was weak for the next few days. When I had recovered enough, I realized that I had no conscious awareness of what had caused my illness. I wasn't aware what the ingredients were in the food I had eaten. There was nothing in my past-life experiences that warned me I had to respond to get the poison out of me and somehow knew that my life might depend on it. However, a very real force of some kind *did know* what was at stake and acted to protect me. Was it some ancient knowledge stored in my genes that had grown out of the past experience of one of my ancestors? Had my genetic memory come to my rescue?

More Evidence that a Life Force Exists

Although research in the area of memory and the paranormal has been going on for years, it is rather haphazard. We do agree upon some facts. As our cells die and we grow new ones, our bodies go through a form of reincarnation. Scientists believe that every seven years all the cells in our bodies are completely replaced. (Remember that our DNA is stable and repairs itself; it isn't replaced over time like the other molecules in our bodies.)

Our Circadian Rhythms

Another interesting biological function is circadian rhythms, which are 24-hour periods or cycles of biological activity or functions in our bodies. Each of us has a 24-hour biological clock. It's located in a tiny region of the brain called the suprachiasmatic nucleus. This clock is affected by light. It controls the rhythms of our bodies throughout the day and night, directing the way our hormones behave and how fast our cells grow daily. Our 24-hour biological cycles may even dictate when we are born.

Studies indicate that more babies are born naturally after midnight than during the afternoon because the birthing clock was set at night. Why does this happen? The answer may also lie deep in our evolutionary past; i.e., a mother and her newborn child in a bygone era would perhaps be in less danger from wild animals and warrior enemies during the night than in the daytime.

Consciousness

Even though our bodies grow from the infantile state to youth, middle age, and old age, our consciousness doesn't change; we remain the same person. Much evidence points to the existence of a conscious energy that exists throughout time. Scientists still can't explain what consciousness is by using the laws of physics and chemistry. But each of us is aware that consciousness exists because we experience it in situations. Question: Does our *genetic memory* reside in this consciousness, or does this consciousness reside in our *genetic memory?*

Reincarnation

Reincarnation is based on the idea that consciousness, life force, or energy (whatever you choose to call it) has existed from the beginning of the human race and can never be destroyed. According to the theory of reincarnation, this energy is *reborn* into human form from time to time.

For centuries, millions of Hindus have held this belief. Reincarnation is also mentioned in the Christian Bible when Jesus is transfigured before his disciples and they ask if he is a reincarnation of an earlier prophet.

In more modern times, Albert Einstein, the physicist famous for creating the theory of relativity, maintained that no energy in the universe is ever lost; that energy only changes its form. This concept may provide some scientific evidence to support the idea of reincarnation. Today, millions of people on this planet believe that individuals are reborn after living one life and may even live a series of lives. Even if you don't believe in reincarnation, the research is interesting, and science hasn't yet been able to prove or disprove the idea.

Past Life Regression

Sometimes, when people are hypnotized or guided to a place of deep memory through meditation, they recall details of previous lives and frequently experience incidents from a possible past life, demonstrating this by speaking in an unfamiliar language. Experts in this field aren't sure whether these people are remembering past lives during past life regression or putting together bits of information they have somehow picked up subconsciously.

Déjà Vu

Déjà vu is French for *already seen*. Sometimes we have the strange feeling of having seen or experienced something before, even though we seem to be seeing or experiencing it for the first time. Scientists don't know what triggers déjà vu. Maybe it's a neurochemical action in our brain when we feel strange and identify the feeling with a memory, even though we are having a new experience. Is it possible we just recall pieces of a true experience and weren't paying complete attention when it happened—so are now filling in the details from some deep well of memory? Or maybe a picture confuses our mind and we think it was a personal event. Was it possibly a story we had heard at a prior time? Some researchers believe that déjà vu may be related to reincarnation, and we may be experiencing something we have already experienced in a previous life.

Other "Footprints" of the Life Force...

As we continue to stalk our genetic memory, we come across other clues about the power of the life force that each of us carries.

A national news story in December of 2003 describes how four New Zealand lifesavers uprighted a capsized delivery truck weighing nearly two tons to free three people trapped inside. Afterward, the rescuers admitted they didn't know how they got the supernatural strength for the rescue.

There are also numerous well-documented stories of people whom doctors expected to die but who waited until a loved one could make it to their bedside or until after the family came together to celebrate a special holiday.

Whatever name you might wish to give it, this powerful life force is working through your genetic memory. Come into harmony with it and you will see your life improve.

Chapter 2—Time Line

The time line helps us understand that over long time frames, as we changed the foods we were consuming, we began to acquire diseases we had never acquired before.

200 Years Ago—No Refined Flour or Rice

During the early 1800s people discovered that if they ground the grain and eliminated the husk it would last longer—but that such treatment removed significant vital nutrients. Flour stayed fresh longer than the grain itself and they could use the flour to bake bread. This process produced white flour, which we all use today. Since bread lasted longer, it would remain on the shelf and increase profits, but it would decrease your health.

The same thing happened with rice. People discovered that when they took off the outside husk of the rice, white rice stayed fresh longer than the brown rice with the husk still on it.

Over time, rich people created recipes for delicious foods made with white rice and white flour. The poor people ate whole grains like brown rice and things made with whole grain flour—and were generally healthy because the husks of the brown rice and whole grains contain most of the vitamins. But the poor people wished to eat like the rich people, and as soon as they could afford it, the poor people began eating white rice and things made with white flour, causing their health to decline. Similarly, the primitive people who enjoyed simple unprocessed foods and started eating the processed foods began to get many of the same diseases.

With the advent of the steel roller mill after the Civil War, the refining process became less expensive and white flour became universally available.

For more than five generations, white flour ground from wheat has supplied the basic ingredient for almost every baked product on American grocery store shelves. The nutrients left us years ago. Now half of the American diet consists of white flour products: bread, cakes, cookies, pastas, pizza, muffins, pies, tortillas, etc.

500 Years Ago—No Potatoes or Rice

(Reprinted from *Potato-History* by W. J. Rayment, with permission.)

- The potato was discovered in the windswept Andes Mountains of South America, a harsh region plagued by rising and falling temperatures and poor soil conditions. Yet the tough and durable potato evolved in its thin air (elevations up to 15,000 feet) and continued to thrive at even higher elevations as the people climbed ever higher on their mountainous terrain.

- Western man did not come into contact with the potato until as late as 1537, when the Conquistadors arrived in Peru. And it was even later, about 1570, that the first potato made its way across the Atlantic to make a start on the continent of Europe.

- Though the potato was productive and hardy, the Spanish put it to very limited use. In the Spanish colonies, potatoes were considered food fit only for the lower classes. When brought to the Old World they would be used primarily to feed hospital inmates.

- It would take over three decades for use of the potato as an edible item to spread to the rest of Europe. The potato was cultivated primarily as a curiosity by amateur botanists. Resistance was due to ingrained eating habits, the potato's reputation as a food for the underprivileged, and perhaps most importantly, its relationship to poisonous plants.

- The potato is a member of the nightshade family and its leaves are, indeed, poisonous. A potato left too long in the light will begin to turn green. The green skin contains a substance called solanine which can cause the potato to taste bitter and even cause illness in humans. Such drawbacks were quickly understood in Europe but not well known in the rest of the world.

- Europe would wait until the 1780s before the potato gained prominence anywhere. At about that time, the people of Ireland adopted the rugged food crop and began cultivating it extensively, primarily for its ability to produce abundant, nutritious food. Unlike any other major crop, potatoes contain most of the vitamins needed for sustenance. Perhaps more importantly, potatoes could be grown in great concentration and so provided sustenance to ten people on a single acre of land. This would be one of the prime causative factors for the Irish population explosion over the following 30 years or so. Of course, by the mid-1800s the Irish would become very dependent upon this crop.

- The early Irish experience with the potato stimulated acceptance for the lowly vegetable throughout Europe.

In France, the potato was imposed upon society by an intellectual, Antoine Augustine Parmentier, who realized that the nutritional benefits of the crop, combined with its productive capacity, could benefit the French farmer. Parmentier was a pharmacist, chemist and employee of King Louis XV. While being held prisoner by the Prussians during the Seven Years War, he was so fascinated by the potato that he decided it should become a staple in the French diet. After his release from prison and an initial failure to convince the French people of its advantages through his writings and speeches, he acquired a miserable and unproductive spot of ground on the outskirts of Paris. There he planted 50 acres of potatoes, hiring a guard to watch over it. This unconventional behavior drew considerable attention in the neighborhood. In the evening the guard allowed the locals to come and see what all the fuss was about. Believing this plant must be valuable, many peasants acquired (stole?) some of the potatoes from the plot and soon were growing the nutritious root in their own garden plots. Thus, resistance was overcome by curiosity and the realization of their desire to better their lot with the obviously valuable new produce.

- Soon the potato would gain wide acceptance across Europe and eventually make its way back over the Atlantic to North America (1719).

1,500 Years Ago—No Refined Sugar

In our human digestive evolution, refined sugar has only been around for a mere "moment" in time. Refined sugar did not exist anywhere in the world until around 500 A.D. In all the eons over which our digestive systems were evolving, the world simply did not have refined sugar—for hundreds of thousands of years. Yet our ancestors survived, even though they lived in harsh physical conditions. In a few places around the world, a little honey or sugar cane may have been available occasionally—but usually to kings and queens only. They were the first people to acquire diabetes in all of human history.

From the beginning, our ancestors did not have the luxury of eating combination foods. They ate like animals eat today; one food at a time, and in a completely unrefined form. The foods and kinds of carbohydrates they ate did not require large amounts of insulin secretion.

For hundreds of thousands of years, our ancestors ate only a low GI diet, and as a result, the pancreas did not have to secrete as much insulin per day (or in their entire life!) as our pancreas has to secrete daily in modern times.

Simple Sugars

The first kind of carbohydrate is a simple sugar. Simple sugars include table sugar, honey, jelly, jam and candy. Colas and other kinds of "soft drinks" contain mostly simple sugars (usually made from corn). Simple sugars provide your body with quick energy, but they don't give you any vitamins or minerals, and they don't provide the good nutrition your body needs daily. Exceptions to this are fruits and fruit juices, which contain vitamins as well as a simple sugar called fructose. Whole fruits, by the way, are even better for you than fruit juices because they have more fiber, which improves health. If you are going to eat simple sugars, choose fruit and eat it in moderation. Read labels. Lots of snack foods, canned items and frozen foods are loaded with sugar. Eating an excess of simple sugars every day causes weight gain and increases the chance of becoming diabetic.

Diabetes, of course, is a disease that can trigger serious effects like infertility, blindness and kidney disease. Medical science has long since proven that obesity is linked to heart disease, some types of cancers, strokes, and numerous other ailments.

Complex Carbohydrates

The second kind of carbohydrate is called a "complex" carbohydrate. Complex carbohydrates are built like many simple sugar molecules linked together. This makes complex carbohydrate molecules bigger than simple sugar molecules. Because their structure is more complicated than simple sugars and their molecules are bigger, it takes your body longer to break down complex carbohydrates into a form it can use for energy. This is good because during this processing, small glucose molecules are gradually released, helping to regulate the level of sugar in your blood. This explains why the energy you get from complex carbohydrates lasts longer than the energy you get from simple sugars. It also explains why you don't experience a "sugar rush" as you do when a large amount of simple sugar quickly enters your bloodstream all at once. Complex carbohydrates come from plants—particularly vegetables and grains. Another name for complex carbohydrates is "starches." Breads, spaghetti, noodles, rice, and pasta are all examples of complex carbohydrates.

If breads or pasta are made from flour that has been refined so that the outer husk of the grain has been removed, they are almost like simple sugars—all energy and no vitamins. All the vitamins were in the outer husk that got taken off and thrown away during the manufacturing process, leaving sugar.

White bread and rolls and white rice are examples of starches that have been refined. Whole grain breads and rolls and brown rice are examples of unrefined starches. Generally, the less processing a grain goes through, the better it is for your body. Even puffing a cereal takes away some of the nutritional value. Plain oatmeal is much healthier to eat. If unrefined grains are so good for us, why do we see so many things made with white flour and why do we eat white rice? Well, as we said earlier, years ago people discovered that refined flour and white rice stayed fresh longer. In our time, scientists often study cultures where poor people eat whole grains and are healthier. The bottom line is: the less a carbohydrate (or any food) processed, the better it is for you. Eat an apple or a piece of celery or a whole grain bagel, and leave the candy bar and the white bread alone.

5,000 Years Ago—FFFVN (Fruit, Fowl, Fish, Vegetables, Nuts)

For 99.9 percent of the time humans have lived on earth, our diets have been comprised of wild game and plants. As a result, our pre-agricultural ancestors consumed fewer calories per mouthful, yet the foods were rich in fiber, vitamins, minerals, and other health-enhancing compounds. Their diets were low in total and saturated fats and high in special fats like omega-3 fatty acids. Their diets were more than just chance. Nutritional Genetics is not just about good health; it is a fundamental part of our evolution.

How do we know what our ancestors ate? Anthropologists have pieced together a fairly clear picture of what our ancestors ate. Their conclusions are based on:

- Archeological evidence;
- Studies of modern day hunter-gatherer populations in Australia, Africa and South America; and

- The nutritional analysis of wild game and plants.

Archeological Evidence

This category of evidence consisted of thousands of ancient human bone fragments, full skeletons, skulls, campsites, weapons, tools, burial graves, carved and engraved objects, paintings, and even footprints that have been unearthed.

Modern Hunter-gatherers

Hundreds of modern day hunter-gatherer societies have been studied. These subjects range from the Aborigines in Australia to southern African tribes, and tropical forest dwellers, such as Pygmies, to tribes in the Philippines and Paraguay and grass-landers from Venezuela.

The variety of foods these people consumed included wild game and uncultivated wild plants, similar to the range of foods our ancestors ate. These tribes are not perfect replicas of the past, but they have lived without technology and offer close approximations of how people survived over time.

Good Genes

We have embraced the idea that because our parents are healthy we are more likely to be free of disease and live longer. This may or may not be true.

First example: Verona Johnson, who was the oldest living American in 2005, lived to be 114 years old. Johnson's father died at sixty-nine; her mother died at eighty-five. Verona ate moderately, and in her final years walked seven flights of stairs every day. Her long life was due to healthy eating and an active lifestyle. She almost certainly did not inherit longevity directly from her parents.

Second example: In 1998, Swedish scientists did a study to prove that shared genes are not the major factor in longevity. The scientists looked at identical twins who had been separated at birth and lived apart from each other to see if the twins died about the same time. They found the average difference in the twins' lifespan could be up to thirty percent. This means that one twin could die at seventy and the other might live to be 100 years old.

Third example: If there are two brothers in a family and one brother lives to be 100, there is a seventeen times greater chance that the other brother(s) will live to be 100, as well. This evidence holds true for sisters at 8.5 times the rate. We believe that these brothers and sisters who were brought up in the same household and shared the same lifestyles allow for these high longevity statistics.

While genetic research on body weight, obesity and aging is still in its infancy, most research shows that lifestyle factors—what you eat, what you do, and how you keep an active mind—have a considerably greater influence on helping you stay lean, healthier, and living longer.

More about Genes

By current estimates, about 30,000 genes in our body spread out across the forty-six chromosomes (twenty-three pairs) and are found in the nucleus of most of our cells. Our genes can instruct our body how to respond to stress, including responses to inadequate amounts of food or too much food. An example of genes that can help or hinder is the body fat and its effect on you in other areas like the human leukocyte antigen (HLA) genes. HLA genes constitute a group of about 150 genes located on chromosome number six (which contains genes that control your body's response to insulin and affect your body fat level, among other functions). They are very important to your overall health. New studies also suggest that the HLA genes may be linked to obesity, coronary heart disease and aging itself.

New studies suggest that it is a combination of your genes, your environment, and your lifestyle that determine your status. If you have an average set of genes (as most of us do), it is your lifestyle that becomes the most important factor in your ability to stay lean and healthy and live to a ripe old age. Having good genes and a healthy lifestyle would be most desirable, but genes are the luck of the draw and beyond our control, at least for now. Lifestyle, on the other hand, is entirely within our control. If you make good choices, you have a better than average chance of staying lean throughout your lifetime.

Sedentary Lifestyle

Unfortunately, recent research reveals that Americans are not very healthy. Despite the unquestioned fact that the United States still ranks number one in technology and science and is among the leaders in healthcare information, it is interesting to note that a recent study by the World Health Organization (a United Nations agency) has ranked the U.S. 24th out of 191 countries for life expectancy.

Why are we Americans ranked so low? Part of the answer may be due to the way we live. Our daily routine consists mainly of getting in the car, driving to work, sitting at a desk—possibly at a computer—and then getting into the car and driving home. Once there, we push more buttons—on the microwave, dishwasher, washer, dryer, television, etc.—until it's time for bed, and the next work day we repeat the cycle. Food is available 24 hours a day, seven days a week, and when it comes to food portions, most Americans have been conditioned to think that "bigger is better."

The future doesn't look promising. Nutrition scientists are already predicting that our children may be the first generation that does not live as long as their parents. Why? The number one vegetable eaten by North American children is French fried potatoes. By the age of three, North American children already have fat deposits in their arteries. Babies born in 2000 have a thirty- to fifty-percent chance of being dangerously overweight and developing diabetes. And diabetes, it has been found, can cause many other diseases, including cancer and heart disease. It can also lead to impotence and blindness, and can result in amputation of limbs. What may be most terrifying is that diabetes can be difficult to detect. People may be in a pre-diabetic state for as long as seven years without even knowing they have it.

Global Epidemic

An increase in obesity is occurring worldwide and becomes more widespread each year, more or less in direct relationship to increases in sugar consumption. From Beijing to Budapest, Helsinki to Barcelona, and Boston to San Diego, scientists are observing near-epidemic rates of obesity in children.

Historically, obesity has been viewed as a cosmetic problem rather than a health issue. We, as healthcare professionals and concerned human beings, must be aware that while infectious diseases used to be the world's greatest health epidemic concern, diabetes is fast becoming the epidemic of the 21st century. There is little evidence, indeed, to contradict the medical opinion that our Western diet is the responsible factor in this developing global pandemic.

Chapter 3—
The Treatment

The Gifts Anomalies Give Us

An anomaly is something that doesn't follow the known rules. It is "something that isn't supposed to happen, but does." Anomalies are situations, circumstances and events that are exceptions to or apparent diversions from the way things usually work.

Scientists often ignore anomalies, but they can be a major source of scientific advancement, because even if something happens only one time in ten million, there *must be* some mechanism to explain how and why the exception happened. By continuing to study genetic anomalies—unexplained phenomena that rarely occur in nature and man—nutrition scientists open the way for discovery of new medicines and drugs that may allow all of us to increase our healthy lifespan.

Penicillin—An Anomaly that Saves Millions of Lives Each Day

Although anomalies are generally ignored, some of our greatest discoveries, like the discovery of penicillin, have resulted from taking a close look at those "exceptions to the rule."

In 1928, at St. Mary's Hospital in London, John Alexander Fleming was researching agents that might fight bacterial infections. One day, as he left for a short vacation, he forgot to wash some of the glass plates upon which he had been growing cultures. When he returned to his laboratory a few weeks later, mold had grown on one of them, but the bacteria he was studying were not growing around the mold. Instead of throwing out the moldy plate, Fleming studied it, developed a reasoning for the occurrence, and discovered penicillin. In 1941, that powerful antibiotic came into general use during World War II and saved thousands of lives and continues to do so today.

Two Modern Anomalies—How They May Help You and Your Children Live Longer, Healthier Lives

Hyaluronic Acid (HA)—Tomorrow's Fountain of Youth

A modern anomaly that may extend your life and the lives of your children is just beginning to be known and studied. It's a substance called *hyaluronic acid,* which your body naturally creates and which decreases in your body as you grow older.

In the U.S., hyaluronic acid has been used in eye surgery as a shock absorber to protect the retina, and it is also used as a lubricant for arthritic joints. More recent studies have also shown that it may help to heal wounds and build new tissue.

Rapid Aging

Two studies are especially important. The first deals with children who have Juvenile Progeria, also known as Hutchinson-Gilford Syndrome. The second study deals with people who have Werner Syndrome, medically referred to as Adult Progeria. People who have either type of Progeria lose a great deal of hyaluronic acid in their urine.

Progeria is a rare but incurable genetic disease. People with Juvenile Progeria carry in their DNA a genetic mutation that speeds up the aging process so much that when they die, at ten to fifteen years of age, they look like old men and women. Although the prevalent cause of death is heart disease, these children do *not* show all the signs of aging. Boys don't develop prostate problems; boys and girls don't get cancer or cataracts. High blood pressure, stroke, diabetes and Alzheimer's disease—all of which are common in normal old age—are rare.

Werner Syndrome begins to develop after puberty. The reproductive organs of people with Werner Syndrome fail to develop normally and completely, and they fall victim to many types of cancer. But, still, diabetes, high blood pressure, stroke, prostate problems, and Alzheimer's disease remain rare, indeed.

Slowing the Aging Process

On the opposite end of the spectrum we can observe people living in the village of Yuzuri Hara, Japan, who enjoy unusually long and healthy lives. About ten percent of the people in the village are over eighty-six years old. They remain very active, and many of them have soft, smooth skin, a condition typical of people much younger. Villagers rarely need a doctor and hardly ever contract cancer, diabetes, or Alzheimer's disease. Their good health and long lives do not seem to be specifically due to a healthy lifestyle; some villagers smoke, and most do not use sun block or skin cream even while working many hours in their fields. The reason for their long, healthy lives seems to lie in their diet, which includes very little meat and lots of homegrown, sticky starches. The hills around the village are not conducive to growing rice. Instead, the villagers grow several different types of potatoes, varieties that are uniformly rich in hyaluronic acid.

As if to prove that their traditional diet creates their good health, those who embrace a western diet are, like others we have mentioned earlier, having problems. From soon after the time at which these villagers began to incorporate western processed food into their diet—a few years ago—heart attacks have doubled. Also, children who move away from this unique area and begin to eat a western diet are now dying long before their elderly parents.

HA seems to provide a key to living a long, healthy life. Essentially, the children with Progeria lose their ability to process hyaluronic acid and begin looking like old people. The long-lived, healthy Japanese villagers thrive, it seems, on the HA in the foods they consumed.

The Power of Diet

More evidence of the impact of diet on health and lifespan comes from recent studies of the American Pima Indians who have lived in Arizona for hundreds of years. Until about 1950, these people were thin, fit, and very healthy. Now they are the second most obese people in the world. Eighty percent of them now have diabetes, and their life expectancy is only forty-seven years.

In stark contrast to the Arizona Pima decline in health status, the Pima Indians who live in Mexico—a people with the same genetic background— continue to be thin, fit, and healthy.

The only significant difference is diet. Those in Arizona consume more food, and it's made with white flour, white sugar, and a lot of fat-laden shortening. They eat a lot, but are not getting good nutrition—which can (and apparently does!) lead to disease.

If you are following the *North American* diet, you are much more likely to suffer debilitating and possibly fatal diseases, and you will die younger than you should.

This way of eating is not confined to the United States and Canada, by the way; studies show that nearly twenty-five percent of Europeans are now eating poorly, as well.

Here is an interesting but puzzling set of facts. Scientists have never found a gene for death; and humans are not genetically programmed to grow progressively weaker, contract diseases and eventually die.

If you can recognize and work with your genetic intelligence, you should be able to live much longer, possibly even to age 100 and beyond, and have perfect health. Is that not something worth thinking about? And during this time of extended lifespan, medical science may be able to work with nature to discover drugs to help extend life expectancy and a high quality of life for all people even more. We may find or be able to create our own internal fountain of youth. Some promising areas are already on the horizon. Next, we will look at some examples.

Walnuts Help Prevent Heart Disease

The walnut has been useful for millennia. The Egyptians used walnut oil to preserve their mummies. Now, pulverized walnut shells are used for a part of the insulating shield in the nose cones of certain rockets in the U.S. space program.

Beyond those historical (and non-nutritional) uses, an exciting new possibility for the walnut has been discovered that can benefit every person on this planet. For the first time in its history, the FDA (Food and Drug Administration) in the U.S. has allowed advertisers to claim that eating 1.5 ounces of walnuts a day, as part of a diet that is low in saturated fat, cholesterol and calories, may reduce the risk of coronary heart disease. Well-researched studies have repeatedly shown that a diet rich in walnuts made arteries as much as sixty-four percent more elastic and reduced the level of molecules that can constrict blood vessels by twenty percent. It also reduced cholesterol levels in the groups that were studied.

Researchers believe that these benefits may be related to the fact that walnuts contain high levels of omega-3 fatty acids, as well as L-arginine and vitamin E. The health community supports these claims, even though the evidence is still preliminary and limited.

As this sort of research moves forward, we are getting closer to discovering other natural medicines found in foods. Ongoing studies suggest that the lycopene found in tomatoes may help prevent prostate cancer, a type of cancer that is expected to strike eighty percent of the male population in North American sometime during their lives.

Apo A-I Milano

Another exciting discovery helped scientists develop a new drug that may reduce the need for artery-clearing surgery. In 1975, a middle-aged man visited his doctor in Milan. The patient's total cholesterol levels were terribly high, and he had a very low level of the good cholesterol. Anyone else with these levels would not be alive. However, the man showed no sign of cardiovascular disease. Researchers at the University of Milan discovered that his parents had lived long lives. They tested his entire village and found that forty other people had the same abnormality. Every individual was descended from the same set of ancestors in a line that began in 1780, and each person had a mutated gene, which scientists named Apo A-1 Milano. No one knows what caused the mutation. Was it something in the soil on that 1780 couple's homestead? Was it something in the water? Or more likely, was it something they ate over the years—and how it was prepared? Preventology can bring hope to millions!

Walk down the halls of any large hospital and you will probably see signs reading: Adolescent Medicine, Cardiology, Child Physiology, Clinical and Metabolic Genetics, Clinical Pharmacology and Toxicology, Endocrinology, Gastroenterology and Nutrition, Hematology/Oncology, Immunology and Allergy, Infectious Diseases, Neonatology, Neurology, Pediatric Medicine, Respiratory Medicine, Rheumatology, Section of Gynecology, Cardiovascular Surgery, General Surgery, Neurosurgery, Orthopedic Surgery, Plastic Surgery, Urology, Clinical Biochemistry, Hematopathology, Microbiology, Molecular Genetics, and Pathology.

But something is missing. Why don't we see a sign for **Preventology** *to protect us in advance from all these possible illnesses so we can have a prolonged, healthy life?* It is because there is no such department, no such specialty, no concentration of effort in the medical community on what is perhaps the broadest field of all—*living life in an all-encompassingly healthy way.* There are only piecemeal efforts within each specialty to provide anecdotal (and often not particularly helpful) advice on things one can do to stave off a specific disease without regard to the larger context of life itself as a frame of reference.

I am proposing an entirely new field of medicine. **Preventology** will help you use natural substances in natural ways to help adapt and alter your lifestyle so you can work with your genetic memory and enjoy the benefits of your intrinsic Genetic Intelligence to produce good health and longer life, beginning today.

And you will be able to accomplish this without the financial strain and worry of buying high-priced drugs or taking expensive medical treatments.

Scientists have now mapped all of the genetic code we are aware of today, and they are working with flatworms and fruit flies to learn more about genes which may be adapted or altered to improve our future lives. Since assured outcomes from these studies and theories remain decades away, why not start now with healthy foods? This is a function of **Preventology.**

If the current work with genes is successful, medical researchers think they will be able to identify genetic markers 75 to 100 years into the future. These markers will be able to diagnose a disease in the early stages, and will be able to minimize its effects even if they possibly can't keep that disease away. But note the undertone in this otherwise rosy and hopeful prediction. Our medical establishment is still focused on attempting to cure diseases, not on preventing them.

Here's an anecdote from my own past. As a young pharmacist working at Johns Hopkins, arguably one of the finest hospitals in the world, I was eager to see what these world-renowned specialists ate to maintain their health. During my break, I followed many of them to the cafeteria to quietly observe what they chose to eat. I was shocked to see these eminent doctors loading up on the same *junk foods,* crammed with sugar and trans-fatty acids, that they warned their patients against eating.

There is no doubt about this: As a society and as members of the world's people we need to change our approach. If we continue to devolve into unhealthy people at the rate we do now, our hospitals will not be able to handle the aging Baby Boomer population.

Another aspect of **Preventology** is this: *Sometimes all it takes to prevent disease and stay healthy is a common-sense approach to exercise.*

The Gifts of Exercise

Centuries and even millennia ago, when the hunting was poor and our hunter-gatherer ancestors had to go without food, their bodies adapted by a slowing of the metabolism. And although we do not experience this phenomenon today because we generally do not need to, this mechanism is still working within us. As evidence that it is—a dieter will sometimes reach a frustrating "plateau" beyond which it is hard to lose additional weight because his or her body metabolism has automatically dropped to conserve energy.

However, over the centuries our bodies have not developed a mechanism to cope with our sedentary lives. Our ancestors were food hunter-gatherers who seldom stopped moving, and our bodies were designed to be active. If we don't get adequate exercise, our health deteriorates.

Moderate physical exercise does wonders for our bodies. It increases the adaptability and maintains the capacity of the heart and lungs, helping to compensate for the effects that aging has on these organs. Physical exertion opens up arteries in the heart muscle, so if one artery becomes blocked, blood will still reach the tissues, thereby reducing the possibility of a heart attack. Exercise also reduces blood pressure, thus minimizing the risk of a stroke. And exercise even helps muscles release stored insulin into the bloodstream so there's less to stimulate the growth of colon cancer or breast cancer. Recent studies have shown that walking briskly for half an hour every day can cut your cancer risk significantly.

I worked at the Veterans Administration Hospital in Delaware for five years. Part of my job consisted of drug counseling for new patients. I could usually tell how old someone was and what diseases he probably was carrying just by looking at him. I recall observing two men who looked to be in their late forties but were really in their late eighties—with no major diseases. When we looked at them, my co-workers and I thought I had the wrong paperwork. I discovered that the only thing different about these two men was that they walked two miles every day, rain or shine.

Perhaps walking two miles a day isn't for you, but how much exercise is enough, and what kind should it be? Good question. Make a note of it.

Exercising too much or too hard *can* be detrimental to your health. Jim Fixx, a well-known and popular advocate for running, died at the relatively early age of fifty-two from a heart attack suffered while he was running. Ironically, he had reported previously to friends that he was experiencing some chest pain and discomfort on earlier runs, but he never did consult a doctor.

The key to effective exercise, therefore, appears to be moderation—and self-awareness. For several decades, from the 1950s until the mid-'80s, Harvard Medical School researchers tracked more than 17,000 male Harvard University graduates to see the effect of exercise on their life spans. The conclusion was that moderate physical activity would likely lengthen life by about two years.

Other studies also show that *voluntary* exercise seems to be more effective in helping people live longer than *mandatory*, *prescribed* exertion. As a practical matter, it's also important to vary the types of exercise (walking, running, stretching, weight training, etc.) and to use as many muscle groups as possible; in sum, to keep your exercise program interesting enough so that you will stay motivated.

It goes without saying (but we'll say it anyway—see the Jim Fixx example above) that it is most important to check with your doctor before beginning an exercise program.

As for the sources you might use to discover and select exercise routines that you will enjoy, there are hundreds of good books and web sites to help you get started.

Exercise doesn't have to be expensive or complicated. Even working in your yard or garden regularly will help.

Physical Fitness vs. Health Fitness

Have you been *screenwashed?*

Today, people view good health as having a physically fit body, and the standard for physically fit is a slender body with a low body weight—even if that is achieved through plastic surgery and liposuction instead of diet and exercise.

As a healthcare professional working in the best hospitals in the United States, I was constantly amazed that people who fit this standard image of health came into our hospitals with a variety of diseases.

Why do you suppose this is true? Think Hollywood. Hollywood—the entertainment industry in general—is the brainwashing capital of the world. The images of slender bodies on movie and TV screens affect society and their ideals without much relationship to reality. I call it being *screenwashed.* *Screenwashing* in television commercials and magazine advertisements also promotes those calorie-rich burgers, fries, pizza, colas and all those foods high in fat and calories. Maybe this is why dieters are constantly confused.

Today we all hear and see a lot about "makeovers." Television promotes people making over their bodies, their professional images, and their homes. Using the principles in this book—*The Cure Code*— you can create and develop your own internal makeover, a makeover that will help prevent disease and prolong life.

Diet—the Best Medicine?

You, Your Emotions and Your Diet

Your mind, emotions and your body are intimately connected. Have you ever grabbed a sweet snack because you were upset about something or you were lonely and food seemed to numb that feeling for the moment?

If you want to improve your diet and keep to your plan, you'll need to understand the reason you are eating. If it's for any other reason than hunger pangs, close the refrigerator door and learn new ways to find comfort.

It's Never Too Late to Change Your Eating Habits

Your body is constantly changing, even if it isn't obvious. Although you can't see it, the process of creation, maintenance and dissolution is constant in every atom in the human body. Scientists have tracked these atoms to see how they are exchanged with the atoms in the environment around you. They have discovered that, every year, ninety-eight percent of the atoms in your body become completely new. This means that a positive change in your eating habits can affect your body, no matter how old you are.

Eat Less, Live Longer

When you eat less, your body temperature and insulin levels drop. The level of 5-Dehydroepiandrosterone (5-DHEA), a hormone that may slow or reverse signs of aging, stops declining. Authoritative studies have shown that this can extend your life span.

The people of Okinawa, as just one example, have the longest life expectancy of anyone on earth; twenty to thirty percent live longer than Americans. They have virtually no heart problems or strokes and fewer hormone-linked cancers than we do in the West. Why? There are many factors: Okinawans don't drink alcohol or smoke, and they eat little meat. Most of their food comes from plants. Just as important, Okinawans stop eating the minute they begin to feel full, something we all should do. Okinawans are not sedentary, and they meditate or turn to strong family and community support when they are under stress instead of using antidepressants, alcohol *or comfort foods*. We know that their genes don't give them long lives, because those who migrate to the west and live as we do have the same lifespan as an average Westerner.

Carbohydrates—Are They Good for You?

Restricting your calories does not mean restricting carbohydrates. Your healthy ancestors ate lots of vegetables, fruits, and some grains that provided few calories but gave them a lot of fiber. These were carbohydrates that are made up of carbon, hydrogen and oxygen. Carbohydrates give you energy. Here is the logic of this: Your body is made of carbon; organic chemistry tells us that the organic compounds that form plants and animals are carbon compounds; and the genetic messengers in your DNA are made up of carbohydrates.

The *right kinds of carbohydrates* are good for you. In your body, carbohydrates burn without leaving any residue. When you restrict carbohydrates in a high-protein diet, your body breaks down your fat reserves and muscle. But when fat and protein are burned, toxic substances called ketones and aldehydes are produced.

Yes, it's all right to eat carbohydrates as long as you choose those with a low glycemic index—the kind that don't raise your insulin levels disproportionately. But if you eat complex carbohydrates and lots of fiber, fill up with whole foods that are rich in antioxidants and that have been processed as little as possible. In this way, you can lower your calorie intake, stay slim, and live longer.

Studies focused on complex carbohydrates like hyaluronic acid may reveal how these substances protect your cells, and how they could help to prolong your life. Remember how the Progeria children, who look like old men and women, lose a great deal of hyaluronic acid in their urine, and how Japanese in the village of Yuzuri Hara, who grow and eat potatoes rich in hyaluronic acid, enjoy unusually long and healthy lives?

Protect Yourself from Free Radicals

Oxygen free radicals—also called "oxidants"—are molecularly "separated" fragments of the oxygen molecule that enter our bodies every day in our food and our air. Our bodies also produce these oxygen fragments as we digest food.

Free radicals are very unstable. By that I mean, in stable molecules, the electrons are paired. These "lonely" oxygen free radicals have an extra electron that seeks stability by searching within the body for an electron to pair up with in other molecules—essentially attacking other molecules in an effort to get that potential partner. The net effect is that these oxygen free radicals damage cells. It is thought that these aggressive free radicals cause damage to our DNA, which is one of the factors that produces aging.

And the way we live determines how much free radicals damage our DNA. For example, too much strenuous exercise can produce a lot of free radicals, and the more free radicals working to "pair up" with DNA molecules, the more the negative impact on your health.

The accumulation of DNA damage also contributes to the development of diseases associated with aging like cancer, heart disease, Parkinson's disease, Alzheimer's, and senility.

Antioxidants Help

Antioxidants help protect your body from free radical damage by providing free radicals the extra electron they seek to bond with. This induced pairing makes the free radicals stable and they stop attacking other molecules that they could really damage.

Over the centuries, your ancestors' bodies developed a complex antioxidant system that protected them from the harm that could be caused by free radicals, germs, viruses and bacteria. The diet of your hunter-gatherer ancestors was naturally rich in antioxidants, and their strong immune systems protected them from disease.

However, when agriculture replaced the hunter-gatherer mode of living, people's diets contained fewer plants that were rich in antioxidants. As a result, their immune systems were not as strong and they contracted more diseases. Today, thanks to highly processed foods and other imbalances in the diet, most people consume only a fraction of the antioxidants found in ancient diets—so much so that it is estimated that only about one out of every hundred people in the United States today eats a diet that contains an adequate amount of antioxidants.

What about Vitamins?

Some people try to make up for this deficiency, as well as other nutritional deficiencies in their diet, by taking vitamins. Although taking vitamins may be beneficial, studies have shown that taking high doses of some vitamins, like vitamin A, can be dangerous. Also, a single study recently conducted on mice at the Lipid Treatment and Research Center at the New York University Medical Center found that antioxidant vitamins increased bad cholesterol, the kind that makes plaque build up in your arteries leading to heart disease. Even if later studies show that taking antioxidant vitamins doesn't increase bad cholesterol in human beings, does taking vitamins really help you stay healthy?

As Dr. Miriam Stoppard points out in her book, *Defying Age: How to Think, Act and Stay Young,* "Food contains micro-nutrients that help our bodies use antioxidants and send them where they're supposed to go—vital ingredients that you won't find in supplements."

If you rely on supplements to make up for the vitamin deficiencies in your diet, you are fooling yourself. You may even be using those pills and capsules as an excuse for not eating properly. At the very least, you are wasting your money. If you feel you must take vitamins, take a good, balanced multiple vitamin, but only after you have included as many vitamin-rich foods in your diet as you possibly can. And don't forget to include foods rich in flavonoids—those powerful antioxidants found in soy and in certain fruits and vegetables that are the topic of endless heath food articles. Look for the deep pigment in foods. The deeper and richer the color, the more antioxidants are present in the fruit or vegetable. For example, the red pigment in tomatoes is called lycopene. Researchers believe lycopene protects men from prostate cancer. Other studies show that a lycopene deficiency possibly makes it more difficult to cope with old age. Nature has given you a pharmacy in her foods. It's up to you to take advantage of it.

Should You Go Vegetarian?

Today, an increasing number of people who want to reduce their consumption of red meat for health reasons are exploring a semi-vegetarian diet.

Although you may not want to become a vegetarian, on the whole, vegetarians appear to be healthier and to live longer than the general American population. This is probably due to consuming more fruits and vegetables than the rest of us.

If you do decide to try a vegetarian diet, make sure you include enough protein. Most vegetarians eat soy products (if they are not allergic to them), and combine foods such as beans and rice to create balanced proteins similar to the protein found in meat. Some vegetarians also eat fish, eggs and/or dairy products.

Vegetarians who do not eat eggs need to find a source of vitamin B-12 so they do not develop a deficiency in their diet. In this case, B-12 supplements may provide a workable solution.

What's Ahead?

In the future, scientists may be able to create drugs to help prevent many diseases. For example, it takes about seven years before a diabetic state is detected. A drug that could detect this developing state and reverse or stop the process would benefit millions of people.

Can We Prevent Aging?

There are more than a dozen major (and often conflicting) theories about the cause of aging, but no one is sure how to prevent or to reverse it. Discovering a gene that will stop or reverse the aging process would be a great breakthrough for mankind. Unfortunately, this is decades away. Now that the human genome has been mapped, work being done on worms and fruit flies may show scientists how to slow your genetic clock, but it may take 75 to 100 years to find the human genes that affect aging. And even when scientists discover these genes, they may not be able to control them.

Will you live long enough for science to solve the mystery of aging? What can you do in the meantime to improve your health and extend your life?

You can lengthen or shorten your life simply by how you live it. For example, in one specific human chromosome, a particular anti-aging feature has been found to be more common in people who live to be a hundred years old or older than it is in the rest of the population However, half of those who live to this extended age don't carry this anti-aging feature, so their lifestyle must be the causative factor, not some passive genetic predisposition.

On the negative side, some research seems to indicate that our bodies wear out because our DNA becomes so damaged over time by our unhealthy lifestyles—and by outside influences such as pollution in our air, water and food—that our genes eventually lose the ability to repair themselves.

The most important information, in this writer's opinion, is that studies show that eating well, exercising regularly, and possibly using vitamins reasonably may all play a part in extending life expectancy.

Remember that the theory of genetic memory states: Somehow you and your body can understand or remember what happened to your ancestors. You can use the theory of genetic memory to work with the genetic intelligence you have received from your great, great grandfathers and grandmothers and reap benefits that will help you prolong your life and minimize the negative effects of aging. But also remember that nourishing the genes you inherited from your ancestors with the wrong foods can cause this beneficial system to break down. Over and over, studies show that when modern hunter-gatherer societies like the Aborigines in Australia or the Ache in Paraguay began to eat a modern diet, their disease rates climbed; and within one or two generations their health status deteriorated to that of the typical North American.

Preventology—The Answer to America's Growing Health Crisis?

The new tools **Preventology** can give you are critical right now because Americans are facing a health crisis unlike any other we have ever experienced. Much of this crisis is being caused by the growing obesity of our population. In the United States, morbid obesity has surpassed both heart disease and cancer as a leading cause of death. Also, obesity is a crucial factor in all the major modern diseases associated with aging.

A similar pattern is emerging in the rest of the industrialized world as people consume more refined foods high in sugar and fat while "enjoying" an increasingly sedentary lifestyle.

On the other hand, we are also beginning to see that those lean, physically fit individuals who pursue exercise to the extreme often die young.

Baby Boomers are rewriting the past in many ways. We are actively searching for a cure to the problem of aging. We want to stay youthful and healthy, and pass on the promise of long and healthy lives to our children and our grandchildren.

Today, most people still believe that age-related diseases are the end of the line on the road to death. But we were never programmed to die. We don't have a gene for death. The concept of **Preventology** puts us on the cutting edge of a new medical age. Like Columbus, we are sailing off into uncharted waters. Queen Isabella and King Ferdinand of Spain made Columbus's voyage possible, and his discovery changed the face of history forever. You are the kings and queens who are supporting our efforts and opening up a bright new future for yourselves, your children and your grandchildren and for generations yet to come.

More Thoughts to Ponder

- Children today may be the first generation that will not live as long as their parents.
- You are acquiring diseases faster and dying younger than you were meant to. Let *The Cure Code* help you discover your internal fountain of youth.
- With *The Cure Code*, you can empower yourself to prevent disease and live a more youthful and longer life.
- With few exceptions, you were never genetically designed to be overweight. Win the battle against obesity for yourself and your children.
- Learn to harness the health power you already possess. Instead of waiting 75 or 100 years for genetic researchers to come up with a cure for aging, empower yourself today. Follow *The Cure Code* to team up with the genetic intelligence that is your birthright—and enjoy a healthy life.

Chapter 4—The Products

One of the oldest binding documents in history is The Hippocratic Oath. Hippocrates, who is considered the father of western medicine, is still held sacred by physicians. He stated that food is the best medicine. I decided to write this chapter based on multiple requests from individuals who attended our seminars. We provided such seminars at the American Diabetic Association, American Cancer Society, and Whole Foods. We always had the same specific request from those who attended. Perhaps it was best stated by a woman who said, "The new and the old food pyramid and many other efforts of healthcare professionals to help maintain a healthy lifestyle have failed. Please help us by giving us something to put in our mouths that makes a difference."

So we created two new products. Please feel free to contact us to help you acquire them. The first product is the Fountain of Youth Pie. The purpose of the Fountain of Youth Pie is to enhance the overall health of people by following the principles of the emerging science of Nutritional Genetics. Our delicious Fountain of Youth Pie is made from Japanese sweet potatoes, which are rich in hyaluronic acid (HA). The theory is that HA cocoons your cells and prevents diseases.

The people from The Village of the Fountain of Youth in Japan have found HA in these sweet potatoes, and rarely have any serious diseases. The older women, even those in their nineties, rarely have aged skin and appear to be wrinkle free.

The following five points of evidence provide further benefits of this product:

- **Okinawans provide further strong evidence**

  Okinawans, who eat Japanese sweet potatoes at each meal, have the longest disability-free life expectancy in the world. They also have the highest percentage of centenarians (people over 100) anywhere on earth. The average life expectancy of men is seventy-eight years and the average women lives to age eighty-six. This healthy lifestyle contributes to twenty percent less heart disease per capita than in the West, twenty-five percent fewer breast and prostate cancers, and nearly thirty-five percent less dementia than in the United States.

- **Recalling Village of the Fountain of Youth**

  Medical researchers believe that the Japanese village Yuzuri Hara, ("The Village of Long Life,") and its residents may hold the key to anti-aging secrets. The local diet that is unique to the village is a responsible agent for good health. Rarely do these people need to see a doctor, and they are rarely affected by cancer, diabetes or Alzheimer's disease. Toyosuke Komori, the town doctor, who has studied and written books on longevity in Yuzuri Hara, believes that locally grown starches (primarily sweet potatoes) help stimulate the body's natural creation of a substance called hyaluronic acid (HA), which aging bodies usually lose, as we mentioned in an earlier section of this book. HA may ward off the aging process by helping the cells of the body thrive and retain moisture, keeping joints lubricated, protecting the retinae of the eyes and keeping skin smooth and elastic. Hyaluronic acid has also anecdotally been shown useful in all three medical disciplines—orthopedics, ophthalmology, and dermatology, particularly in Asia. Western experts are skeptical, though, about its positive effect when taken in pill form.

These long-lived healthy Japanese villagers, and the Okinawans who eat Japanese sweet potatoes as the core of every meal, consume HA in their foods and live long healthy lives. The theory is that HA cocoons the cells and helps to prevent disease.

- **Progeria Children (specific genetic benefit)**

  Progeria Children Syndrome is an extremely rare incurable, genetic disease, which causes premature, accelerated aging. Progeria ages the body rapidly leaving teens with frail bodies and causing early death. Hyaluronic acid seems to provide a key to living a longer, healthier life. Essentially the children with Progeria lose their HA, looking like old people. What these children lost, these people found. The long-lived healthy Japanese villagers and Okinawans who eat Japanese sweet potatoes as the core of every meal consume HA in their foods and live long healthy lives. The theory is that HA cocoons the cells and prevents disease.

- **Restylane—HA is already present in our bodies**

  Restylane contains hyaluronic acid (HA) and is a crystal clear gel that is a component of the body's own lubricant fluid. HA is plentiful in our bodies when we are born; it is found in all human connective tissue. HA also occurs naturally in the deep layers of our skin (the dermis). It helps to keep skin smooth and tight through its ability to hold up to 1,000 times its weight in water. This natural component holds moisture and may be the secret to youthful, healthy, vibrant skin.

As we age, our bodies produce less and less HA, causing our skin to lose its elasticity and allowing lines and wrinkles to develop. Healthy, youthful skin comes from the inside, and by replacing the components that naturally deplete with age; we have the ability to reverse the signs associated with aging.

- **Suppress appetite**

  The fiber of sweet potatoes provides a feeling of fullness and satisfaction. A number of people have validated the magic of the Japanese sweet potato and have testified to how it has affected them in positive ways. Here are just a few examples.

  - One man who always came home for dinner with a huge appetite had eaten the Japanese sweet potato pie hours prior to returning home. He had absolutely no appetite for the dinner his wife had prepared.

  - A golfer, who always had a huge appetite after playing golf, had also eaten the Japanese sweet potato pie prior to his round of golf and still had a feeling of fullness and loss of appetite hours later.

  - A couple that visited a buffet on a regular basis and the lady realized her appetite wasn't there for a big meal and couldn't take advantage of the buffet. The

Japanese sweet potato pie had suppressed her appetite from earlier in the day.

The sweet potato pie also contains complex carbohydrates, protein, vitamin A and C, iron and calcium, ranking highest in nutritional value.

Because the sweet potato is high in antioxidants, vitamin E and beta-carotene, it is a good source of dietary fiber. It lowers the risk of constipation, diverticulitis, colon and rectal cancer, heart disease, diabetes and obesity. The sweet potato is a great food choice for diabetics to avoid glucose.

The North Carolina Stroke Association, American Cancer Society and the American Heart Association all endorse the theory of sweet potatoes as a nutritious food.

The Second Product is Resvera Juice

This product has no sugar added. It is sweetened with agave. (Which comes from a cactus). It is FDA-approved as a sweetener for diabetic patients.

This information is supported through research by medical professionals at the Harvard Medical School.

The following four points show the benefits of this product.

Heart Disease–French Paradox

- The French Paradox refers to the fact that people in France suffer relatively low incidence of coronary heart disease, despite their diet being rich in saturated fats. It is shown that France's high consumption of red wine is the primary factor in this trend. The red wine that is consumed has a compound known as resveratrol, which may help reverse complications of obesity, which could extend life.

Alzheimer's Disease
- Studies show that resveratrol lowers the levels of amyloid-beta peptides, which are amino acids that are the main component of plaque in the brains of Alzheimer patients.

Cancer
- The natural compound, resveratrol, found in grapes, mulberries, peanuts, and other plants and food products, including red wine, may protect people from cancer and cardiovascular disease. It acts as an antioxidant, anti-cancer and anti-inflammatory. It also has a positive effect on cholesterol levels.

Stimulation of Longevity Genes (Specific Genetic Benefit)
- **Resveratrol stimulates 1,000 of your longevity genes.** Harvard biologist David Sinclair published results of experiments in the 2003 journal *Nature*. He concluded that resveratrol significantly extends the lifespan of the yeast, Saccharomyces cerevisiae. Dr. Sinclair also founded Sirtris Pharmaceuticals to promote resveratrol or related compounds as anti-aging drugs.

  The author observed resveratrol supplementation with foods extends lifespan and delays motor and cognitive age-related decline in the prevention of aging-related diseases in the human population. This confirms that resveratrol must trigger our natural genetic defenses against aging.

The Solutions
The Cure Code is working in the emerging new science of nutritional genetics. The educational component in this book,

along with seminars, will provide one of a two-part solution to provide health and longevity.

The first component—education, will help individuals understand that as we changed the nutritional time line in which we began to eat foods that mankind had never eaten before, such as refined sugar, refined flour, potatoes, rice and combination meals, it changed the genetic time line. Most importantly it caused us to acquire diseases that we never had before such as diabetes, cancer, heart disease and many others.

The second component is food products. These new types of food will continue to expand and improve the arsenal we have created and help us to combat disease. Our children are the first generation that will not live as long as their parents. If we don't change the foods that we eat, the lifespan of Americans will begin to decrease. So please join us in using the *The Cure Code* to help provide solutions to these life-threatening problems.

Please feel free to contact me at **www.TheCure-Code.com**

Selected References

Appleby, Julie. "Health Insurance Premiums Crash Down on Middle Class." *USA Today.* 17 March, 2004, sec. B:1.

ARA Content. "Preventing Childhood Obesity: What Parents Can Do." 22 March 2004. Fitness & Kids. *<http://www.fitnessandkids.com/preventing-childhood-obesity.html>.*

Austad, Steven. *Why We Age.* New York: J. Wiley & Sons, 1997. (p. 201)

Carroll, Tobert Todd. "déjà vu." The Skeptic's Dictionary. 30 Dec. 2003. *<http://skepdic.com/dejavu.html>.*

"Cleaning Up Clogged Arteries." *Reader's Digest.* April 2004:29.

Chopra, Deepak, M.D. and Simon, David, M.D. *Grow Younger, Live Longer: 10 Steps to Reverse Aging.* New York: Random House, Inc., 2001.

Chopra, Deepak, M.D. *Perfect Health: The Complete Mind Body Guide.* New York: Three Rivers Press, 2000.

"Cookbook Advice: Eat Walnuts, Live longer!" 9 Dec. 1998. *<http://www.news.wisc.edu/wire/i120998/walnuts.html>.*

"The Discovery of Penicillin." Nobel e-Museum. 26 May 2003. The Official Website of The Nobel Foundation. *<http://www.nobel.se/medicine>.*

Ducasse, C. J. "The Case of the Search for Bridey Murphy," *A Critical Examination of the Belief in Life After Death, Part 5, Chapter 25.* The International Survivalist Society, Articles. *<http://www.survivalafterdath.org/articles.htm>.*

Fabrishnikov, Major I. I., M.D., Ph.D. "Complex Inherited Recollections." 11 April 2004. *<http:// IllyaArticles/COMPLEX_INHERITED_RECOLLECTIONS.htm>.*

Fabrishnikov, Major I. I., M.D., Ph.D. "Complex Inherited Recollections." 11 April 2004. <http:// IllyaArticles/Hypnotic_Regression.htm>.

Gardner, Amanda. (HealthDay Reporter.) "Walnuts a Smart Choice for the Heart." 26 March 2004. *<http://healthfinder:gov/news/newsstroy:asp?docID=518095>*. [Sources: Emilio Ros, M.D., head, Lipid Clinic, Hospital Clinic of Barcelona, Spain; Marc Siegel, M.D., clinical associate professor, medicine, New York University School of Medicine, New York City; March 23, 2004, *Circulation*, online.]

Holmes, Richard. Past Life Memories and Experiences. *<http://geocities.com/richard_holmes/reincarnation/how-people-remember.htm>*.

Hyman, Mark, M.D. and Liponis, Mark, M.D. *Ultraprevention*. New York: Scribner, 2003:151–152.

Kaufman, Marc. (Washington Post Staff Writer.) "FDA to Allow Claim of Health Benefits for Walnuts." 1 April 2004; Page A02. *Washingtonpost.com*. *<http:www.washingtonpost.com/wp-dyn/articles/A40651-2004Mar31.html>*.

Klatz, Dr. Ronald and Goldman, Dr. Robert. *Stopping the Clock: Longevity for the New Millennium*. North Bergen, New Jersey: Basic Health Publications, Inc. 2002, 22-24; 175–207.

Marchand, Lorraine H. "Obesity Associated with High Rates of Diabetes in the Pima Indians." *The Pima Indians: Pathfinders for Health*. Obesity and Diabetes. National Diabetes Information Clearinghouse. *<http://diabetes.niddk.nih.gov/dm/pubs/pima/obesity/obesity.htm>*.

McConnaughey, Janet (Associated Press). "Diabetes Warning for Children." 22 March 2004. Fitness & Kids. *<http://www.fitness and kids.com/kids-diabetes.html>*.

Michel, Karen (producer). "Genetics of Aging and Longevity: Search for the Fountain of Youth." Unraveling the Mysteries of Genetic Science. The DNA Files, SoundVision Productions. (On Air beginning Nov. 2001.) *<http://www.dnafiles.org/about/pgm13/>*.

"The Mystery of Consciousness." Coming Back: The Science of Reincarnation. 13 Jan. 2004. *<http://www.mantra-mediation.com/science-reincarnation.html>*.

O'Sullivan, Matt and McLean, Robyn. "Rescuers Flip Van to Safety." National News Story. 30 Dec. 2003 *<http://www.stuff.co.nz/stuff/0,2106,2757029a11,00.html>*.

"Progeria." Diseases and Conditions. 15 Dec. 2003. *<http://www.manbir-online.com/diseases/progeria.htm>*.

Province, Charles M. "George S. Patton, Jr., U.S. Army, 02605, 1885-1945." The Patton Society's Website.*< http://www.geocities.com/pattonhq/homeghq.html>*.

Pyle, Encarnaclon. "Holding on to Life: Patients Seem to Defy Science." *The Columbus Dispatch*. 2 Jan. 2004.

Ratey, John J. *A User's Guide to the Brain*. New York; Pantheon Books, 2001. (p. 188)

Rayburn, Julie S. "Why are We Killing Our Children?" 22 March 2004. Fitness & Kids. <http://www.fitnessandkids.com/art_our_childrn.html>.

Rayment, W.J. "Potato-History." Copyright 2000–2010.

Ross, Emma and Verrengla, Joseph B. (Associated Press Reporters.) "Too Much Latitude: Epidemic of Obesity Becomes A Worldwide Killer." *The Columbus Dispatch.* 9 May, 2004: Insight, B3.

Somer, Elizabeth, M.A., R.D. *The Origin Diet: How Eating Like Our Stone Age Ancestors Will Maximize Your Health.* New York: Henry Holt and Company LLC, 2001.

Somers, Suzanne. *Fast & Easy.* New York: Crown Publishers, 2002, 22–26; 33-38; 40-44.

Somers, Suzanne. *Get Skinny on Fabulous Food.* New York: Random House, Inc., 1999.

Steward, H. Leighton, Bethea, Morrison C., M.D., Andrews, Sam S., M.D. and Balart, Luis A., M.D. *The New Sugar Busters!* New York: Ballantine Books, 2003, 31–32; 62–74.

Stoppard, Dr. Miriam. *Defying Age; How to Think, Act and Stay Young.* First American Edition. New York: DK Publishing, Inc., 2004.

"The Village of Long Life." *abcNEWS.com.* [Reprinted from a synopsis of an article which appeared on ABC's 20/20 show featuring Connie Chung.] 21 March 2004 <http://www.humanbodyrecon.com/fountain.html>.

Wells, Donna. "Overcoming Childhood Obesity." *Columbus Parent.* March 2004, 19–20.

Yang, Sarah. "The Power of Circadian Rhythms." WebMD*Health*, Feature Archive. 8 May 2000. <http://my.webmd.com/content/article/11/1674_50522>.